ZOHRA FTAITI

Vegan Body Revival: Ignite Your Wellness And Achieve Weight Loss Through The Power of Plant-based Living

Unlocking Vibrant Health And Sustainable Weight Loss With Whole foods

Copyright © 2024 by Zohra Ftaiti

All rights reserved. No part of this publication may be reproduced, stored or transmitted in any form or by any means, electronic, mechanical, photocopying, recording, scanning, or otherwise without written permission from the publisher. It is illegal to copy this book, post it to a website, or distribute it by any other means without permission.

The information provided in "Vegan Body Revival: Ignite Your Wellness and Achieve Weight Loss Through the Power of Plant-based Living" is for general informational and educational purposes only. The contents of this book are not intended to serve as a substitute for professional medical advice, diagnosis, or treatment. Readers are advised to consult a qualified healthcare professional before making any health-related decisions or for guidance about a specific medical condition.

First edition

This book was professionally typeset on Reedsy.
Find out more at reedsy.com

This book is lovingly dedicated to my baby brother Mourad, whose vegan journey transformed not just his health but also inspired this book. Through embracing plant-based living, he's become a beacon of vitality and proof that profound health and energy are rooted in what we eat. This work is a tribute to his journey, aiming to empower others with insights, research, and recipes for a vibrant, sustainable life. Here's to embracing change and inspiring transformation.

Contents

Introduction to Vegan Body Revival: Ignite Your Wellness and... 1
Chapter 1: The Foundations of Vegan Nutrition 3
Chapter 2: Debunking Vegan Myths 12
Chapter 3: The Path to Wellness: Holistic Health and... 18
Chapter 4: Vegan Weight Loss Strategies 26
Chapter 5: Healing from the Inside Out 32
Chapter 6: Building Strength and Stamina 40
Chapter 7: Transitioning to Veganism 47
Chapter 8: Meal Planning and Prep 52
Chapter 9: Recipes for Revival 57
Chapter 10: Sustaining Your Vegan Lifestyle 72
Conclusion: Your Vegan Body Revival 79

Introduction to Vegan Body Revival: Ignite Your Wellness and Achieve Weight Loss Through the Power of Plant-based Living

Welcome to a journey of transformation, where the path to wellness and sustained weight loss is not just about what you eat, but how you live. "Vegan Body Revival" is more than a book; it's a mission to redefine your relationship with food, health, and the environment. Written from a place of deep understanding and personal experience, this guide is designed to illuminate the power of plant-based living in a world where diet culture often dominates our choices.

The inspiration behind this book stems from a simple yet profound realization: that the foods we choose to nourish our bodies can either be the most powerful form of medicine or the slowest form of poison. Through these pages, you'll discover the science and soul of vegan nutrition—how a diet rooted in whole foods and natural ingredients can ignite your wellness, revitalize your energy levels, and help you shed weight sustainably.

But this book goes beyond the basics of vegan eating. It delves into the myths and misconceptions that often surround plant-based diets, armed with evidence-based research and real-world success stories. From debunking the protein myth to exploring the environmental impact of our food choices, "Vegan Body Revival" is a comprehensive guide to understanding the why's and how's of veganism.

As we embark on this journey together, you'll learn not just about the nutritional foundations of a vegan diet, but also about the holistic approach to wellness that it embodies. This includes stress management, sleep hygiene, and the integration of exercise and mindfulness into your daily routine. Each chapter is meticulously crafted to equip you with the knowledge, strategies, and recipes you need to transform your health and embrace a lifestyle that's kind to your body and the planet.

So, whether you're a seasoned vegan looking to deepen your knowledge, or a newcomer curious about the benefits of plant-based living, this book is for you. It's a call to action—a chance to join the movement of individuals choosing health, vitality, and sustainability. As we turn the page to the next chapter, get ready to embark on a life-changing adventure that promises not just a healthier body, but a renewed sense of purpose and well-being.

Moving into the next chapter, "Foundations of Vegan Nutrition," prepare to delve into the core principles that make a vegan diet both nourishing and fulfilling. We'll explore the essential nutrients vital for optimum health, debunk common myths, and provide practical advice on assembling balanced, nutrient-rich meals that support both body and mind. This chapter is not just about what to remove from your diet but about discovering the abundance of foods that promote healing, energy, and longevity. Join us as we continue on this journey, uncovering the building blocks of a diet that doesn't just feed the body but nourishes the soul.

Chapter 1: The Foundations of Vegan Nutrition

Macronutrients and micronutrients in a vegan diet.

Embarking on the "Foundations of Vegan Nutrition" chapter, we delve into a treasure trove of plant-based nourishment, spotlighting the key players in the vegan nutrient lineup. This detailed exploration not only uncovers the essentials of a balanced vegan diet but also equips you with a menu of power-packed foods and their nutritional profiles.

Macronutrients

First up, macronutrients—the big guys. We're talking proteins, carbs, and fats. The common question here is, "Where do you get your protein?" Spoiler alert: plants have plenty. We'll explore how legumes, grains, nuts, and seeds are not just protein-rich but also packed with energy-sustaining carbs and healthy fats. It's all about finding the right balance to keep your engine running smoothly.

In the journey through vegan nutrition, understanding the sources of macronutrients is pivotal. Let's delve into the proteins and fats that are fundamental to a vegan diet, ensuring you're not just eating but thriving on plant-based goodness.

Proteins are the building blocks of life, essential for building and repairing tissues, making enzymes, and more. For vegans, abundant sources include:

1. **Seitan**: A chewy, protein-rich food made from gluten, ideal for mimicking the texture of meat in various dishes.
2. **Tofu, Tempeh, and Edamame**: Soy products offering a complete protein profile, versatile in cooking from scrambles to stews.
3. **Lentils**: Packed with protein, fiber, and minerals, perfect for soups, salads, and sides.
4. **Beans:** Including varieties like black, pinto, and kidney beans, great for adding heft to meals.
5. **Nutritional Yeast:** A cheesy-flavored condiment, providing not only protein but also vitamins B12 and B6.
6. **Quinoa and Buckwheat**: Whole grains that serve as complete proteins, excellent in salads or as side dishes.
7. **Chia Seeds and Hemp Seeds:** Seeds that offer a good protein punch and can be easily added to smoothies, yogurts, and baking.

Fats, equally crucial, provide energy, support cell growth, and help absorb vitamins. Vegan sources include:

1. **Chia Seeds and Flaxseeds:** Rich in ALA, a type of omega-3 fatty acid, beneficial for heart health.
2. **Coconut Oil and Olive Oil**: Healthy oils for cooking and dressing, rich in medium-chain triglycerides and monounsaturated fats, respectively..
3. **Nuts and Nut Butters:** Almonds, walnuts, and cashews are not just

protein-rich but also good sources of healthy fats

4. **Avocados**: A versatile fruit loaded with monounsaturated fats, perfect for salads, sandwiches, or as a creamy base for dressings
5. **Cacao Nibs**: A delightful source of antioxidants and fats, adding a chocolatey crunch to snacks and desserts

Carbohydrates: The energy currency of the body, found in:

1. **Whole Grains**: Such as brown rice, barley, and oats, offering a sustained energy release.
2. **Fruits and Vegetables**: Especially berries, oranges, and leafy greens, packed with vitamins, minerals, and fiber.

By incorporating these protein, carbohydrate and fat sources into your vegan diet, you ensure a rich intake of essential nutrients, paving the way for a balanced, healthful lifestyle that supports your body's needs. As we journey further into the realms of whole foods and balanced plates, remember that variety is the spice of life—and of optimal health.

Micronutrients

Now, onto the micronutrients. These are the unsung heroes of your diet, crucial for everything from bone health to brain function. We'll dive into how a kaleidoscope of fruits, vegetables, and whole grains can cover your nutritional bases, ensuring you're not just surviving on a vegan diet but thriving.

Micronutrients, vital for optimal health, are nutrients required by the body in smaller amounts but are crucial for development, disease prevention, and well-being. Vegan diets, while abundant in many micronutrients, may require attention to certain nutrients to ensure adequacy and prevent deficiencies.

1. **Vitamin B12**: Essential for nerve function, DNA production, and red blood cell development. Vegan sources are limited, necessitating fortified foods or supplements. Deficiency can lead to anemia and neurological issues.
2. **Iron:** Integral for oxygen transport in the blood and muscle function. Plant-based sources include lentils, beans, tofu, and fortified cereals. However, iron from plant sources (non-heme iron) is less readily absorbed than that from animal products (heme iron), making it important for vegans to consume vitamin C-rich foods to enhance absorption.
3. **Calcium:** Crucial for bone health and vascular function. Vegan sources include fortified plant milks, tofu made with calcium sulfate, and leafy green vegetables. Adequate intake helps prevent osteoporosis.
4. **Vitamin D**: Supports bone health and immune function. Few foods naturally contain vitamin D, making fortified foods and sunlight exposure important. Supplements may be necessary, especially in areas with limited sun exposure4 source.
5. **Zinc**: Important for immune function and wound healing. Vegan sources include legumes, nuts, seeds, and whole grains. As phytates in plants can inhibit zinc absorption, techniques like soaking beans, fermenting, and choosing leavened grain products can enhance its bioavailability.
6. **Omega-3 fatty acids**: Essential for brain function and heart health. ALA (alpha-linolenic acid) is a plant-based omega-3 found in flaxseeds, chia seeds, hemp seeds, and walnuts. Conversion rates of ALA to EPA and DHA (more active forms of omega-3) are low in humans, so algae-based supplements might be considered.
7. **Iodine:** Vital for thyroid function, which regulates metabolism.

Iodized salt and seaweed are vegan sources, but intake levels should be monitored to avoid deficiency or excess.

8. **Selenium**: Plays a role in antioxidant defense and thyroid hormone metabolism. Brazil nuts are a potent source, with just one or two providing the daily requirement. Other sources include whole grains and legumes.

Ensuring a well-planned vegan diet that includes a variety of these foods, possibly supplemented by specific nutrients, can help maintain optimal health and prevent micronutrient deficiencies.

The Importance of Whole Foods

Whole foods are the unsung heroes in the narrative of health, playing a pivotal role in maintaining and enhancing our well-being.

Emphasizing whole foods in a vegan diet is not just about eliminating animal products; it's about prioritizing the healthiest versions of plant-based foods. Whole foods, including vegetables, fruits, whole grains, legumes, nuts, and seeds, are minimally processed, retaining most of their natural fiber, vitamins, minerals, and other beneficial compounds. Here's how focusing on whole foods can have practical and beneficial impacts on your health and daily life:

1. **Nutrient Density:** Whole foods provide a high nutrient-to-calorie ratio. They deliver essential vitamins and minerals without the added sugars, fats, and preservatives found in processed foods. For example, choosing a whole apple over apple-flavored snacks not only reduces sugar intake but also increases fiber, vitamin C, and phytonutrients.

2. **Natural Fiber**: The fiber in whole foods, such as beans, lentils, and whole grains, supports digestive health and can help maintain a healthy weight. Fiber keeps you feeling full longer, reducing the temptation for unhealthy snacking and aiding in weight management.
3. **Heart Health:** Whole foods are key in managing blood pressure and cholesterol levels. Diets rich in fruits, vegetables, and whole grains have been linked to a reduced risk of heart disease
4. **Blood Sugar Management:** The complex carbohydrates in whole foods digest more slowly than refined grains and sugars, leading to more stable blood sugar levels. This is especially beneficial for preventing and managing diabetes.
5. **Environmental Impact**: Emphasizing whole foods minimizes your environmental footprint. Whole foods require less packaging and processing than their processed counterparts, contributing to less waste and lower greenhouse gas emissions.

To make whole foods a practical part of your daily diet, consider these tips:

- **Stock your kitchen** with a variety of fruits, vegetables, whole grains (like quinoa and brown rice), and legumes (such as lentils and chickpeas).
- **Plan meals around whole foods**, starting with a vegetable or grain base and adding flavors with herbs, spices, and plant-based proteins.
- **Prepare in bulk** to save time, cooking grains and legumes in large quantities to use throughout the week.
- **Snack on whole foods**, choosing nuts, seeds, and fresh fruit over processed snack foods.

By focusing on whole foods, you're not just following a vegan diet; you're

CHAPTER 1: THE FOUNDATIONS OF VEGAN NUTRITION

choosing a lifestyle that promotes optimal health, sustainability, and a more mindful way of eating.

But how do we artfully balance a vegan plate with these whole foods? Picture your plate as a canvas, with each color representing a nutrient essential to your body's well-being. Half of this canvas should be painted with a variety of vegetables and fruits—vibrant greens, deep reds, and sunny yellows—ensuring a rich intake of vitamins, minerals, and antioxidants. A quarter should be dedicated to whole grains like quinoa, barley, and brown rice, providing you with fiber and energy. The remaining quarter is reserved for protein-packed legumes, nuts, and seeds, building blocks for your muscles and brain.

Balancing a Vegan Plate with Whole Foods

Crafting a balanced vegan plate is akin to painting a masterpiece with a palette of nature's finest hues. It's not just about the colors but about creating a harmonious blend that nourishes your body and delights your senses. Here's how to turn each meal into a nutritious work of art:

Half of Your Plate: Vegetables and Fruits

Start with a rainbow of vegetables and fruits. Think leafy greens like spinach and kale, offering iron and calcium; bright bell peppers and carrots, packed with vitamin C and beta-carotene; and blueberries and strawberries, bursting with antioxidants. This isn't just about aesthetics; it's a way to ensure you're getting a wide range of nutrients. Aim for at least three different colors to maximize the variety of vitamins and minerals.

A Quarter of Your Plate: Whole Grains

Whole grains are your energy canvas. Quinoa, not just a grain but a complete protein, barley with its heart-healthy fiber, and brown rice, rich in B-vitamins, lay the foundation of your meal. They're not just fillers; they're fuel, offering sustained energy and supporting digestive health.

A Quarter of Your Plate: Proteins

Legumes like black beans, lentils, and chickpeas; nuts such as almonds and walnuts; and seeds like flaxseeds and chia seeds are the protein strokes on your canvas. They don't just build and repair muscles but are also vital for brain health and energy metabolism.

Practical Tips for a Balanced Vegan Plate

- **Experiment with Herbs and Spices**: Elevate the flavors of your plate with a sprinkle of fresh herbs or a dash of spices. Not only do they add zero calories, but many herbs and spices are also packed with antioxidants.
- **Incorporate Healthy Fats:** A drizzle of olive oil on your vegetables, a slice of avocado on the side, or a sprinkle of hemp seeds over your salad introduces healthy fats necessary for absorbing fat-soluble vitamins.
- **Stay Hydrated**: Complement your meal with water, herbal teas, or freshly squeezed juices to aid digestion and nutrient absorption.
- **Plan Ahead:** Prepping ingredients in advance can make assembling your colorful plate both quick and enjoyable. Cook grains in bulk, chop veggies for easy access, and have a variety of canned or cooked legumes ready to go.

CHAPTER 1: THE FOUNDATIONS OF VEGAN NUTRITION

By viewing each meal as an opportunity to nourish your body with a spectrum of whole foods, you're not just eating—you're curating a vibrant array of nutrients that work in concert to support your health and well-being.

Alright, let's turn the page from all those colorful plates of whole foods and dive headfirst into the sea of myths and tall tales. Chapter 2, "Debunking Vegan Myths," is where we roll up our sleeves and get down to business, cutting through the haze of misunderstandings surrounding the vegan way of life. Picture this: a journey packed with hard facts and heartfelt stories, lighting up the real deal about vegan eats and their powerhouse role in keeping us and the planet thriving.

Now that we've got the lowdown on what makes a vegan diet tick, we're more than ready to face off against the myths muddying the waters. Chapter 2, "Busting Vegan Myths," is our map to navigate through the jungle of misconceptions, spotlighting the solid truths that let us rock a plant-based lifestyle with total confidence. It's time to tackle these myths head-on, breaking them down piece by piece, to show off just how kickass vegan nutrition really is.

Chapter 2: Debunking Vegan Myths

Alright, Chapter 2, "Debunking Vegan Myths," is where we gear up for a deep dive into the sea of skepticism that floats around vegan nutrition. We're not just skimming the surface with the usual suspects like protein, calcium, and iron. Oh no, we're going full detective mode on the myths that question whether plant-based diets can really give us all the nutritional jazz we need and celebrate the diversity on our plates.

This chapter is like the myth-busting squad of the vegan world. It's where we pull back the curtain on the biggest misconceptions and give you the lowdown on what's what. We're tackling everything from "Can you even lift, bro?" to "But where do you get your iron?" and everything in between. It's time to squash the rumors that vegan diets are all lettuce and sadness. Spoiler alert: they're not.

So, buckle up, because we're about to embark on a journey filled with science-backed facts, nutrition know-how, and a dash of sass. This chapter is your vegan myth-busting toolkit, ready to arm you with the knowledge to navigate the plant-based life with confidence. Let's debunk these vegan myths together, one truth bomb at a time.

Addressing common misconceptions about protein, calcium, and iron

In debunking the common misconceptions surrounding protein, calcium, and iron in a vegan diet, it's crucial to illuminate how plant-based sources of these nutrients are not only on par with their animal-based counterparts but also bring to the table a plethora of additional health benefits.

Protein: The myth that vegans struggle to meet their protein needs is pervasive yet unfounded. Plant-based proteins like lentils, chickpeas, black beans, quinoa, tofu, and seitan not only provide ample protein but also contain fiber, vitamins, and minerals absent in animal proteins. For example, lentils pack about 18 grams of protein per cooked cup, along with significant amounts of iron, fiber, and folate, contributing to heart health and aiding digestion without the cholesterol found in meat

Calcium: Similarly, the belief that dairy is the only reliable source of calcium is a misconception. Many plant-based foods, such as kale, bok choy, fortified plant milks, almonds, and tahini, are rich in calcium. Broccoli and fortified plant milks not only offer calcium but also provide vitamin K and magnesium, which are essential for bone health. These sources promote calcium absorption without the saturated fat present in dairy products

Iron: Lastly, the concern over iron is easily addressed with a variety of vegan foods rich in this essential mineral. Foods such as spinach, lentils, chickpeas, pumpkin seeds, and fortified cereals are excellent sources. Pairing these with vitamin C-rich foods like bell peppers, oranges, or strawberries enhances iron absorption, tackling the myth that vegans are iron-deficient. This way, vegans can achieve their iron intake while also benefiting from the antioxidants and vitamins present in these foods

Expanding on the importance of prioritizing nutrient-rich plant-based foods, it's clear that adopting a vegan diet allows individuals to not only meet but often exceed their nutritional needs, effectively debunking myths surrounding potential deficiencies in protein, calcium, and iron. Beyond these core nutrients, a vegan diet also offers an abundance of other essential vitamins and minerals critical for maintaining health and preventing disease.

Vitamin B12: Often cited as a nutrient of concern for vegans, B12 can be adequately obtained from fortified foods like plant milks, breakfast cereals, and nutritional yeast, or through supplements, ensuring proper nerve function and blood formation.

Omega-3 Fatty Acids: Crucial for brain health, omega-3s can be found in flaxseeds, chia seeds, hemp seeds, and walnuts, as well as in algae-based supplements, offering a plant-based alternative to fish oil.

Vitamin D: Essential for bone health, vitamin D can be absorbed through sun exposure, fortified foods, or supplements. Mushrooms exposed to sunlight also provide a natural plant-based source of vitamin D.

Zinc: Important for immune function, zinc is abundant in legumes, nuts, seeds, and whole grains, with pumpkin seeds being particularly high in this nutrient..

By incorporating a diverse range of whole, plant-based foods into their diets, vegans can enjoy a wide spectrum of health benefits, including improved heart health, lower risks of chronic diseases, and a lower environmental footprint, all while ensuring their nutritional needs are fully met.

The science behind vegan nutrition and disease prevention

Scientific evidence highlights how a well-planned vegan diet reduces the risk of developing chronic diseases such as heart disease, type 2 diabetes, and certain cancers, thanks to its high content of fiber, antioxidants, and phytonutrients.

The science underlying vegan nutrition and its role in disease prevention is increasingly supported by robust research. A well-planned vegan diet, rich in fiber, antioxidants, and phytonutrients, plays a pivotal role in mitigating the risk of several chronic conditions.

Heart Disease: Vegan diets are linked to a lower risk of heart disease, primarily due to their emphasis on whole grains, nuts, fruits, and vegetables, which are known to lower blood pressure and improve heart health. These foods are abundant in soluble fiber and plant sterols, which can reduce cholesterol levels and decrease the risk of heart disease.

Type 2 Diabetes: By favoring plant-based foods over processed options and animal products, vegan diets can help maintain a healthy body weight, improve insulin sensitivity, and reduce the risk of type 2 diabetes. Foods high in fiber, such as legumes and whole grains, are particularly effective in regulating blood sugar levels.

Certain Cancers: Consuming a variety of fruits, vegetables, and legumes, which are staples of a vegan diet, may also help protect against certain types of cancer. These foods offer a rich supply of antioxidants and phytochemicals that combat inflammation and reduce oxidative stress, factors that contribute to cancer development

By integrating a wide range of plant-based foods, we can harness these nutritional benefits, supporting not only their overall health but also contributing to the prevention of chronic diseases. This approach emphasizes the power of diet in shaping health outcomes and underscores the effectiveness of vegan nutrition in fostering long-term well-being.

Busting the myth of expensive vegan diets

The misconception that vegan diets are inherently more expensive than diets including meat and dairy is widespread yet unfounded. By focusing on whole foods, seasonal produce, and bulk buying, a vegan diet can be both economical and accessible, debunking the myth of high costs associated with plant-based eating.

Whole Foods: Opting for whole foods like grains, beans, vegetables, and fruits, especially when purchased in bulk, can significantly reduce grocery bills. These staples of a vegan diet are not only more affordable than processed vegan alternatives but also offer superior nutritional value.

Seasonal Produce: Purchasing fruits and vegetables that are in season not only ensures that you're getting the freshest produce possible, but it also tends to be more cost-effective. Seasonal buying supports local farmers and reduces transportation costs, which can translate into savings for the consumer..

Bulk Buying: Bulk purchases of staples like rice, lentils, and nuts can lead to significant savings. Many health food stores offer bulk bins where shoppers can buy the exact amount they need, reducing waste and cost. Additionally, many dry goods have a long shelf life, making them ideal for stocking up and saving money over time.

By making informed choices and focusing on the nutritional and economic benefits of whole, plant-based foods, we can enjoy a rich, diverse, and healthful vegan diet without breaking the bank. This approach not only makes healthy eating more achievable for everyone, regardless of budget but also fosters a sustainable lifestyle that benefits both personal health and the environment.

Through these explorations, "Debunking Vegan Myths" not only equips You with factual counterarguments to common misconceptions but also empowers You to make informed decisions about your health and diet, backed by the latest scientific research and practical advice.

Chapter 3: The Path to Wellness: Holistic Health and Lifestyle Choices

Alright, let's dive headfirst into the lush, green world of plant-based goodness, where the perks go way beyond just what's on your plate. This chapter isn't just about counting calories or nutrients; it's about painting a bigger picture of how munching on plants can be a game-changer for your mind, mood, and overall mojo.

We're talking a full-blown exploration into how swapping steaks for kale and quinoa can not only spruce up your physical health but also sharpen your mental edge, soothe your soul, and maybe even give you that zen vibe you've been searching for. With a mix of hard-hitting science and down-to-earth tips, we'll guide you through the ins and outs of living la vida vegan.

From how plant-based munching can be your ally in the battle against the bulge, to its role in keeping your heart ticking like a well-oiled machine, we're covering all bases. But it doesn't stop there – we're also spotlighting the mental perks, like how this diet can be a dynamo for your brainpower and an elixir for your emotions. Plus, we'll throw in some pro tips to make the transition as smooth as avocado on toast.

So, gear up for a deep dive into the world of vegan living, where you'll come out the other side not just informed, but inspired to embrace the green side with open arms (and an eager fork). Let's unravel the power of plants together, one leafy bite at a time.

How plant-based eating influences physical health, mental clarity, and emotional well-being

A well-planned vegan diet is rich in nutrients, fiber, and antioxidants, contributing to improved physical health by lowering the risk of chronic diseases, enhancing digestive health, and promoting a healthy weight. Moreover, the diet's high content of vitamins and minerals plays a crucial role in optimizing mental clarity and emotional well-being. Studies have shown that plant-based diets can improve mood and cognitive function, thanks to their high levels of phytonutrients and absence of the inflammatory properties found in animal products.

Nutrients and Physical Health

Plant-based diets are rich in essential nutrients that play key roles in maintaining and enhancing physical health. These diets provide high levels of vitamins, minerals, and phytochemicals that support bodily functions, improve the immune system, and reduce inflammation. For example, the high content of vitamin C in fruits and vegetables boosts the immune system, while magnesium, found in nuts and seeds, is essential for muscle and nerve function.

Fiber and Digestive Health

The fiber content in plant-based diets is significantly higher than that in diets containing meat and dairy. Fiber aids in digestion by promoting bowel regularity and feeding the beneficial bacteria in the gut microbiome. This not only enhances digestive health but also contributes to the prevention of gastrointestinal disorders.

Antioxidants and Chronic Disease Prevention

Antioxidants present in plant-based foods, such as flavonoids in berries and carotenoids in carrots, combat oxidative stress and reduce the risk of developing chronic diseases, including heart disease, type 2 diabetes, and certain cancers. These compounds neutralize harmful free radicals, protecting cells from damage.

Mental Clarity and Emotional Well-being

The benefits of a plant-based diet also extend to mental health. Phytonutrients and the absence of inflammatory properties found in animal products contribute to improved mood and cognitive function. Diets high in fruits, vegetables, nuts, and seeds are linked with lower rates of depression and anxiety, enhancing overall emotional well-being. The anti-inflammatory effects of plant-based diets can positively affect the brain, leading to increased mental clarity and focus.

In conclusion, by prioritizing plant-based foods rich in nutrients, fiber, and antioxidants, individuals can enjoy enhanced physical health, digestive wellness, and a reduced risk of chronic diseases. Moreover, the mental and emotional benefits, including improved mood and cognitive function, underscore the holistic advantages of embracing a plant-based diet.

How vegan diets support heart health, diabetes prevention, and more

The adoption of vegan diets has been closely associated with numerous health benefits, particularly in the context of heart health, diabetes prevention, and overall metabolic well-being. One of the critical elements of vegan diets contributing to these benefits is the emphasis on unsaturated fats, predominantly found in plant-based foods. These unsaturated fats, including both monounsaturated and polyunsaturated fats, play a vital role in lowering cholesterol levels, reducing blood pressure, and improving blood sugar control, thereby mitigating the risk factors associated with cardiovascular diseases and type 2 diabetes.

Unsaturated Fats and Heart Health

Unsaturated fats, found in abundance in nuts, seeds, avocados, and olive oil, are instrumental in improving heart health. Unlike saturated fats prevalent in animal products, unsaturated fats help lower the levels of harmful LDL cholesterol in the bloodstream, thus reducing the risk of heart disease. Studies have demonstrated that plant-based diets, rich in these healthful fats, can significantly lower cardiovascular disease risk by improving blood lipid profiles.

Diabetes Prevention

Regarding diabetes prevention, the high unsaturated fat content in vegan diets is beneficial for blood sugar control. Foods rich in these fats improve insulin sensitivity, which is crucial for managing and preventing type 2 diabetes. The fiber in plant-based diets also plays a supportive role, stabilizing blood sugar levels and preventing spikes after meals.

Overall Wellness

The benefits extend beyond heart health and diabetes prevention. Diets rich in unsaturated fats from plant sources also contribute to reduced blood pressure and are linked with lower rates of obesity. The anti-inflammatory properties of these fats further enhance physical well-being, playing a role in preventing chronic conditions and promoting longevity.

In summary, the shift towards a vegan diet, focusing on the intake of unsaturated fats from plant-based sources, offers a comprehensive approach to improving heart health, preventing diabetes, and fostering overall metabolic health. This dietary pattern, emphasizing whole foods and minimizing processed items, ensures a nutrient-rich, balanced intake conducive to long-term well-being.

The importance of sleep and stress management

In conjunction with a nutritious diet, adequate sleep and effective stress management are pivotal for holistic health. Plant-based diets can influence sleep quality positively, as many vegan foods are rich in nutrients that promote relaxation and better sleep. Stress reduction techniques, such as mindfulness and meditation, complement the physical benefits of vegan nutrition, enhancing overall well-being and resilience.

Incorporating stress reduction techniques like mindfulness and meditation into a lifestyle that includes a plant-based diet can significantly enhance overall well-being and resilience. These practices work synergistically with the physical health benefits of vegan nutrition to create a holistic approach to health.

Sleep and Stress Management

Adequate sleep is crucial for reducing stress levels. It lessens anxiety by preventing overwork of the heart, allows the brain to recharge, and ensures the body can react appropriately to daily stressors. Stress management techniques, including mindfulness interventions, have shown positive impacts on reducing stress and improving mental health outcomes.

Mindfulness and Meditation

Mindfulness and meditation promote mental clarity and emotional stability, complementing the physical health benefits of a vegan diet. These practices encourage a moment-to-moment awareness of our thoughts, emotions, and sensations, which can lead to healthier food choices and a more mindful approach to eating.

Enhancing Overall Well-being

Together, a plant-based diet, adequate sleep, and effective stress management support a robust framework for health. They contribute not only to lowered risk of chronic diseases but also to improved cognitive function and emotional well-being. By managing stress and ensuring enough rest, we can enhance the nutritional benefits of veganism, fostering a greater sense of well-being and resilience against life's challenges.

In summary, the integration of sleep and stress management techniques with vegan nutrition creates a comprehensive approach to health that addresses both the body and mind. This holistic approach supports heart health, diabetes prevention, and more, demonstrating the interconnectedness of diet, mental health, and lifestyle choices in promoting overall wellness.

Integrating exercise and mindfulness into your plant-based journey

Switching to a plant-based diet isn't just about tweaking your menu; it's about overhauling your whole vibe—mixing up your grub with a hefty side of mental wellness, a dash of getting active, and a sprinkle of staying mindful. It's this whole-package deal that sets you up for a life that's not only healthier but downright richer, all while vibing with the heart of vegan living.

Are you tossing some good old-fashioned exercise into your green-eating mix? That's like hitting the health jackpot. It boosts everything from your muscles to your mood, cranking up your energy and clearing your mind. When you sync up moving your body with chowing down on nature's finest, you're not just eating differently—you're living differently. It's about feeding your soul as much as your stomach, making every step and every bite part of a bigger picture of well-being.

Health Benefits of Exercise

Exercise plays a critical role in improving cardiovascular health, increasing muscle strength and endurance, and promoting flexibility and balance. A plant-based diet supports these physical benefits by providing the body with essential nutrients, antioxidants, and energy, while exercise helps in optimizing the body's use of these nutrients.

Moreover, combining exercise with a vegan diet can lead to better weight management by increasing metabolism and reducing body fat more effectively than diet or exercise alone. This synergy between diet and physical activity also enhances mental health by reducing symptoms of depression and anxiety, improving mood, and boosting self-esteem.

Mindfulness and Exercise

Incorporating mindfulness practices such as yoga into your exercise routine can further deepen the connection between mind and body, enhancing the spiritual aspect of wellness that often accompanies a plant-based lifestyle. Mindfulness exercises, along with physical activities, encourage a more conscious and appreciative relationship with food, promoting eating habits that are aligned with personal health goals and environmental sustainability.

By weaving exercise and mindfulness into their plant-based journey, people can embrace a holistic wellness path that feeds the body, hones the mind, and uplifts the spirit. This approach cultivates a richer quality of life and overall well-being.

Chapter 4: Vegan Weight Loss Strategies

The main idea revolves around the profound impact of plant-based diets on both physical health and mental well-being. Research increasingly supports the notion that diets rich in plant-based foods can offer comprehensive health benefits, significantly beyond just nutritional intake. These benefits encompass a wide array of physical health improvements, including but not limited to, enhanced cardiovascular health, reduced risk of chronic diseases such as diabetes and certain types of cancer, as well as contributions to maintaining a healthy weight and digestive system.

Moreover, the mental health benefits associated with plant-based diets are noteworthy. Emerging studies highlight a positive correlation between plant-based eating and mental health outcomes, including improved mood, reduced symptoms of depression and anxiety, and overall enhanced quality of life. The nutritional components of a plant-based diet, such as increased fiber, beta carotene, and vitamin K, alongside the high levels of antioxidants and phytonutrients, are thought to play a critical role in these health benefits. These dietary components can lead to lower inflammation levels, better nutrient absorption, and overall improved body functioning, which in turn can influence brain health and emotional well-being.

In essence, transitioning to a plant-based diet not only supports physical health by reducing the risk of various chronic diseases and promoting a healthy body weight but also contributes to mental clarity and emotional stability. This holistic approach to health underscores the interconnectedness of diet, physical health, and mental well-being, presenting plant-based eating as a comprehensive lifestyle choice for improved overall health.

Understanding the Role of Calories and Nutrient Density

Understanding the role of calories and nutrient density is fundamental in navigating a vegan weight loss journey. Calories provide the energy that our bodies need to function, but not all calories are created equal. Nutrient-dense foods pack a large number of vitamins, minerals, fiber, and phytonutrients into a relatively small number of calories. These foods not only support weight loss by promoting a feeling of fullness and reducing overall calorie intake but also enhance overall health.

Foods that exemplify this balance include:

- **Vegetables and fruits:** Rich in fiber, vitamins, and minerals, they help in weight management by keeping you fuller for longer. Leafy greens, berries, and citrus fruits are particularly nutrient-dense.

- **Whole grains**: Foods like quinoa, barley, and whole wheat provide essential B vitamins, fiber, and a moderate amount of protein. They offer sustained energy release, aiding in weight management and digestive health.

- **Legumes**: Beans, lentils, and peas are high in protein and fiber, contributing to satiety, reducing cravings, and supporting muscle maintenance during weight loss.

- **Nuts and seeds:** Though higher in calories, they are rich in healthy fats, proteins, vitamins, and minerals, making them a nutrient-dense choice that supports heart health and weight control when consumed in moderation.

By prioritizing these foods, You can enjoy a varied and satisfying diet that supports weight loss goals without compromising nutritional intake, showcasing the importance of choosing foods based on their nutrient density rather than calorie content alone.

Effective Meal Planning and Portion Control for Weight Loss

Effective meal planning and portion control are key strategies for weight loss, especially within a vegan diet. By focusing on the quantity and quality of food consumed, individuals can manage caloric intake without compromising nutritional needs. Here are practical examples to guide meal planning and portion control for weight loss:

1. **Use Smaller Plates for Meals**: Opting for smaller plates can visually trick the brain into feeling satisfied with less food, aiding in portion control without feeling deprived.
2. **Incorporate Measuring Cups and Scales**: Initially, use measuring cups or a kitchen scale to get a real sense of portion sizes. For example, a serving of cooked quinoa is typically ½ cup, which can be precisely measured to avoid overeating
3. **Plan Your Meals**: Spend time each week planning your meals. This ensures a balanced intake of nutrients and prevents impulsive eating. For example, planning a week's worth of breakfasts might include oatmeal with fresh fruit, vegan yogurt with nuts and seeds, and smoothies packed with greens and plant-based proteins
4. **Focus on High-Fiber Foods**: Incorporate plenty of vegetables, fruits, whole grains, and legumes into your meals. These foods

are not only nutrient-dense but also high in fiber, which promotes satiety. A meal example could be a large salad with leafy greens, chickpeas, a variety of vegetables, and a sprinkle of seeds, dressed with lemon juice and a teaspoon of olive oil.
5. **Practice Mindful Eating**: Pay attention to your body's hunger cues and eat slowly to allow your brain to register fullness. Avoid distractions like eating in front of the TV, which can lead to overeating.
6. **Portion Snacks Beforehand**: Instead of eating directly from a bag or box, portion out snacks into small containers or bags. This could mean dividing a bag of almonds into portions of about 23 almonds, which is roughly a one-ounce serving.
7. **Stay Hydrated:** Sometimes, thirst is mistaken for hunger. Drinking water before meals can help control appetite and portion sizes.

By implementing these meal planning and portion control strategies, people following a vegan diet can effectively manage their weight while ensuring they receive all necessary nutrients for optimal health.

Integrating a Physical Activity

Incorporating physical activity into daily routines is essential for overall health and complements the benefits of a vegan diet. Tailoring activities to fit individual fitness levels and preferences ensures sustainability and enjoyment, which are key for long-term adherence. Here are some guidelines to help integrate physical activity effectively:

1. **Start with Achievable Goals:** Begin with activities that match your current fitness level. If you're new to exercise, consider starting

with brisk walking, yoga, or light cycling for 10-15 minutes a day, gradually increasing the duration as your fitness improves.
2. **Incorporate Variety:** To prevent boredom and promote all-around fitness, include a mix of cardiovascular exercises, strength training, and flexibility workouts. Cardio could be jogging or swimming, strength training could include body-weight exercises like push-ups and squats, and flexibility exercises could involve yoga or Pilates.
3. **Find Activities You Enjoy**: Enjoyment is key to consistency. Whether it's dancing, hiking, or martial arts, engaging in physical activities that you look forward to will make exercise feel less like a chore and more like a rewarding part of your day.
4. **Make It Social**: Exercise can be more enjoyable and motivating when done with friends or in a group setting. Consider joining a fitness class, sports club, or scheduling regular exercise meet-ups with friends3 source.
5. **Set Realistic Expectations**: Understand that progress takes time. Set realistic, incremental goals to avoid discouragement. Celebrate small victories to stay motivated.
6. **Listen to Your Body**: Pay attention to how your body responds to different activities and adjust accordingly. Rest when needed, and avoid pushing through pain to prevent injuries
7. **Schedule It:** Treat your exercise time like any other important appointment. Scheduling it into your day can help ensure you prioritize physical activity.
8. **Utilize Technology:** Fitness apps and online workout videos can provide guidance and inspiration, making it easier to workout at home or on the go.

By following these guidelines, you can find the knowledge and tools needed to effectively navigate weight loss within a vegan lifestyle,

CHAPTER 4: VEGAN WEIGHT LOSS STRATEGIES

emphasizing that a holistic approach to health can lead to lasting changes.

Chapter 5: Healing from the Inside Out

Welcome to the chapter that could very well be your game-changer. We're diving deep into the art and science of detoxifying and rejuvenating your body, all through the power of plants. It explores how incorporating plant-based foods into one's diet can not only detoxify the body but also significantly enhance overall wellness.

Through a blend of scientific evidence and practical advice, this chapter serves as a roadmap for those seeking to heal their bodies and minds through the power of plant-based nutrition. It is a testament to the fact that food can indeed be medicine, capable of healing us from the inside out.

Detoxifying Your Body with Plant-Based Foods

Detoxifying your body with plant-based foods is about leveraging the natural power of whole foods to cleanse and rejuvenate your system. Foods that are rich in antioxidants, fiber, vitamins, and minerals play a critical role in supporting the body's detoxification processes. These foods include:

1. **Leafy Greens:** Spinach, kale, and chard are packed with chlorophyll,

which aids in purifying the blood and boosting detoxification.
2. **Cruciferous Vegetables**: Broccoli, cauliflower, and Brussels sprouts contain glucosinolates, which help in liver detoxification.
3. **Berries**: Rich in antioxidants, berries such as blueberries, strawberries, and raspberries help neutralize free radicals and support liver health.
4. **Citrus Fruits**: Lemons, oranges, and grapefruits enhance the body's detoxifying capabilities by promoting liver enzyme function and providing vitamin C.
5. **Beets**: High in antioxidants and other nutrients, beets support liver health and increase the production of detoxification enzymes.
6. **Garlic**: Known for its detoxifying properties, garlic stimulates liver enzymes and helps flush toxins from the body.
7. **Ginger**: This root supports digestion and can help cleanse the body by stimulating digestion and circulation.
8. **Turmeric**: Contains curcumin, which is believed to stimulate bile production in the liver, enhancing detoxification.
9. **Legumes:** Beans, lentils, and peas are high in fiber, aiding in the elimination of toxins through the digestive tract.
10. **Whole Grains**: Quinoa, brown rice, and oats are not only fiber-rich but also support healthy liver function and promote the excretion of toxins.

Incorporating these plant-based foods into your diet can significantly enhance your body's natural detoxification systems, helping to cleanse your body of toxins and promote overall well-being

Healing Recipes and Foods that Promote Wellness and Reduce Inflammation

In the realm of healing and wellness, inflammation is the hidden flame that can either fuel our body's repair processes or, when unchecked, wreak havoc on our health. The key to turning down the heat? A strategic arsenal of anti-inflammatory recipes, each a blend of science, simplicity, and the art of flavor. Let's dive into a curated selection of dishes that embody this balance, turning every meal into a step toward healing.

For those looking to rejuvenate their body and mind with plant-based nourishment, here are some detoxifying recipes that not only cleanse but also pack a punch of flavor and nutrients:

1. **Turmeric & Ginger Tea**: Kickstart your day with this powerhouse duo. Turmeric, with its active compound curcumin, and ginger, both boast anti-inflammatory properties. Steep fresh turmeric and ginger root in boiling water, add a twist of lemon and a dash of black pepper to enhance curcumin absorption, and sip your way to wellness.
2. **Omega-3 Rich Chia Pudding**: Chia seeds are not only rich in omega-3 fatty acids but also in fiber and antioxidants. Mix with your choice of plant-based milk and a touch of maple syrup. Refrigerate overnight for a pudding that fights inflammation while pleasing the palate.
3. **Kale & Quinoa Salad**: A vibrant blend of kale, quinoa, avocados, and an assortment of colorful vegetables. Drizzle with a dressing of extra-virgin olive oil and apple cider vinegar for an anti-inflammatory feast that's as nutritious as it is delicious.
4. **Broccoli and Almond Soup**: Broccoli, a cruciferous vegetable rich in sulforaphane, pairs with almonds, loaded with vitamin E and

healthy fats, to create a creamy soup that's both healing and hearty.

5. **Berries & Beet Smoothie:** Combine the antioxidant power of berries with the detoxifying properties of beets. Add a scoop of plant-based protein powder for an extra boost, blending it all with almond milk for a smoothie that's as anti-inflammatory as it is energizing.

For those looking to rejuvenate their body and mind with plant-based nourishment, here are some additional detoxifying recipes that not only cleanse but also pack a punch of flavor and nutrients:

6. **Golden Turmeric Smoothie**: Blend together bananas, fresh turmeric root, ginger, a dash of black pepper (to enhance turmeric absorption), a spoonful of almond butter, and almond milk. This smoothie is not just a detox powerhouse but also a creamy delight.

7. **Green Detox Soup**: Simmer broccoli, spinach, celery, and garlic in vegetable broth. Once tender, blend until smooth. Season with salt, pepper, and a squeeze of lemon juice for a comforting bowl that detoxifies and nourishes.

8. **Kale and Berry Salad:** Toss fresh kale leaves with mixed berries, sliced avocado, and walnuts. Dress with a vinaigrette made from olive oil, lemon juice, and a touch of maple syrup. This salad is rich in antioxidants and healthy fats, making it perfect for a detox meal.

9. **Quinoa and Black Bean Stuffed Peppers:** Fill halved bell peppers with a mixture of cooked quinoa, black beans, corn, chopped tomatoes, and spices. Bake until the peppers are tender. This dish provides a fiber-rich, protein-packed meal that supports detoxification and sustained energy.

10. **Beet and Carrot Juice**: Juice fresh beets, carrots, an apple, and a piece of ginger for a refreshing drink. Beets and carrots are known for their liver-cleansing properties, making this juice an excellent detox choice.

11. **Sweet Potato and Lentil Curry**: Cook lentils and cubed sweet

potatoes in coconut milk with curry powder, turmeric, and cumin. Serve this hearty curry with brown rice or quinoa for a satisfying meal that's full of detoxifying spices and fiber.

These recipes are designed to support your body's natural detoxification processes, reduce inflammation, and provide a nutritional boost. Enjoy these delicious, plant-based options as part of your journey towards a healthier, more vibrant self.

Each of these recipes embodies the principle that food is more than sustenance; it's a form of medicine. By incorporating these anti-inflammatory meals into your routine, you're not just eating—you're healing, one delicious bite at a time.

Special Focus on Meal Prep, Quick Meals, and Healing Foods

By planning ahead and choosing ingredients that are both nourishing and healing, you can ensure that your plant-based diet is not only beneficial for your health but also manageable on your busiest days.

Incorporating plant-based foods into your diet can be both nourishing and convenient with the right meal prep strategies. Here are practical tips for preparing quick, nutritious meals that support wellness and healing:

1. **Healing Foods:** Focus on incorporating anti-inflammatory foods that promote healing and wellness. Turmeric, ginger, berries, leafy greens, and nuts are all excellent choices. A turmeric ginger tea or a smoothie bowl topped with berries and nuts can serve as both a healing and energizing start to your day.

2. **Batch Cooking**: Spend a portion of your weekend preparing large batches of staples like quinoa, brown rice, beans, and roasted vegetables. These can serve as the base for various meals throughout the week, saving you time and ensuring you have healthy options on hand.
3. **Smart Snacking**: Prepare healthy snacks in advance to avoid reaching for less nutritious options when you're hungry. Ideas include hummus with sliced veggies, fruit with a handful of nuts, or whole-grain crackers with avocado.
4. **Quick and Nutritious Breakfasts**: Overnight oats or chia seed pudding can be prepared in mason jars for an easy, on-the-go breakfast. Just add your favorite plant-based milk, a sweetener if desired, and top with fresh fruits or nuts in the morning.
5. **Use a Slow Cooker or Instant Pot**: These kitchen gadgets are perfect for making soups, stews, and curries with minimal effort. Simply add your ingredients in the morning, and you'll have a warm, comforting meal ready by dinner time..
6. **Sheet Pan Meals**: Roast a combination of your favorite vegetables and a protein source like tofu or tempeh on a single sheet pan for an easy, one-pan dinner. Season with herbs and spices for added flavor.

By incorporating these strategies, you can enjoy delicious, plant-based meals that promote healing and wellness without spending hours in the kitchen. These tips make it easy to maintain a nutritious diet, even on your busiest days.

The Long-Term Benefits of Sticking with a Plant-Based Lifestyle

Adopting a plant-based lifestyle goes beyond the temporary trend; it's a profound commitment to enhancing your health and well-being. The immediate benefits—increased energy, improved digestion, and weight management—are just the beginning. In the long term, the advantages compound, offering a robust shield against numerous chronic conditions.

Long-Term Health Benefits

Heart Health: A plant-based diet is linked to a lower risk of heart disease. The emphasis on whole grains, nuts, fruits, and vegetables naturally leads to a reduction in cholesterol and blood pressure levels, contributing to a healthier heart

Diabetes Prevention: By favoring fiber-rich foods over processed options, a plant-based lifestyle can help regulate blood sugar levels, reducing the risk of developing type 2 diabetes

Cancer Risk Reduction: Certain plant-based foods contain phytochemicals that may lower the risk of developing various types of cancer. By focusing on a diet rich in fruits and vegetables, you're providing your body with antioxidants that combat cell damage.

Weight Management: Plant-based diets are typically lower in calories and higher in fiber, helping individuals maintain a healthy weight over time. This, in turn, reduces the risk of obesity-related diseases

Longevity: Adopting a plant-based diet can contribute to a longer life. By reducing the risk of developing chronic diseases and promoting overall health, individuals can enjoy a higher quality of life for a longer duration.

Mental Health: Emerging research suggests that plant-based diets may also have a positive impact on mental health, reducing symptoms of depression and improving overall emotional well-being.

Recent studies highlight that adopting a plant-based diet can significantly enhance mental health. Specifically, it has been linked to a decrease in depression and anxiety levels and an overall boost in emotional wellness. This improvement is attributed to the diet's high content of antioxidants, fiber, and phytonutrients, which play a crucial role in balancing neurotransmitters and reducing inflammation, a known contributor to mood disorders

Immediate Improvements

Energy Level: Shifting to a plant-based diet can lead to an increase in energy due to the high nutrient density of whole, unprocessed foods.

Digestive Health: The high fiber content in plant-based foods supports digestive health and can alleviate issues like bloating and constipation.

Skin Health: The vitamins and minerals found in fruits and vegetables can contribute to clearer, more radiant skin.

Embracing a plant-based lifestyle is not just about the foods you eat; it's about making a conscious decision to prioritize your health and the environment. The benefits are vast and varied, offering both immediate and long-term advantages that can lead to a more vibrant, healthier life.

Chapter 6: Building Strength and Stamina

This is the chapter where we dive deep into vegan fitness, a domain where the power of plant-based nutrition meets the rigor of physical training. Our focus is twofold: muscle gain and endurance, realms often questioned within vegan athleticism. We debunk myths and lay out a blueprint for thriving on a vegan diet while reaching, and even surpassing, fitness milestones.

First, we tackle **vegan fitness,** shedding light on how to optimize muscle gain and endurance through a plant-centric lens. This section is not just about dispelling doubts; it's about showcasing the potent potential of plants in fueling strenuous workouts and accelerating recovery, setting the stage for a robust physique and enduring stamina.

Transitioning into **workout plans that complement a vegan diet**, we bridge nutrition with action. Here, specific exercise routines are tailored to harness the nutritional benefits of a vegan diet, ensuring that every rep, run, or ride is backed by optimal fueling strategies. This synergy amplifies gains, pushing the boundaries of what's achievable on a plant-based regimen.

Lastly, we delve into **nutritional strategies for enhanced recovery**

Recovery is where the real magic happens; it's where muscles rebuild stronger and stamina expands. We detail how a vegan diet, rich in anti-inflammatory foods and essential nutrients, can drastically reduce downtime and elevate the recovery process, making every training session count.

Together, these key aspects form a holistic view of vegan fitness, illustrating that a plant-based lifestyle is not only compatible with athletic excellence but can be the cornerstone of achieving peak physical condition.

Vegan Fitness: Optimizing Muscle Gain and Endurance

In the space of vegan fitness, optimizing muscle gain and endurance centers around a well-structured nutritional foundation. A plant-based diet, rich in diverse protein sources, micronutrients, and properly timed nutrient intake is crucial for maximizing workout results and ensuring effective recovery.

Diverse Protein Sources

Plant-based diets provide a variety of protein sources essential for muscle repair and growth. Unlike some misconceptions, plant proteins like soy, quinoa, and hempseed offer complete protein profiles comparable to animal sources. These proteins support the body's muscle synthesis and repair processes necessary after rigorous workouts.

Essential Micronutrients

Micronutrients, including vitamins and minerals found abundantly in plant-based foods, are vital for energy production, oxygen transport, and antioxidant defense mechanisms. For example, iron and vitamin B12, crucial for energy levels and endurance, can be optimized through fortified plant-based foods and supplements. Additionally, antioxidants from fruits and vegetables help reduce oxidative stress and inflammation, leading to quicker recovery.

Properly Timed Nutrient Intake

Timing of nutrient intake is pivotal in a vegan athlete's diet. Consuming carbohydrates and proteins shortly after exercise can significantly impact muscle recovery and glycogen replenishment. Plant-based diets rich in whole foods provide both immediate and sustained energy sources and enhance recovery time, allowing athletes to maintain consistent training intensity.

In summary, a well-planned plant-based diet, emphasizing a variety of protein sources, micronutrient balance, and strategic nutrient timing, equips athletes with the necessary tools for optimal performance and recovery, underpinning the comprehensive benefits of vegan nutrition in fitness.

Workout Plans That Complement a Vegan Diet

For individuals following a vegan lifestyle, aligning workout routines with dietary choices is essential for maximizing results and ensuring proper recovery. Here are specific examples of workout routines that complement a vegan diet, focusing on both resistance training and cardiovascular exercises:

Workout plans that complement a vegan diet focus on balancing resistance training and cardiovascular exercises, tailored to meet the unique recovery needs and energy demands of individuals following a plant-based lifestyle. Here are specific examples of workout routines:

Resistance Training

Resistance training is crucial for building muscle on a vegan diet. A balanced routine could include:

Bodyweight Routine: Incorporate exercises like push-ups, squats, lunges, and planks. These can be done anywhere, requiring no equipment, making them ideal for vegans focusing on whole-body strength without added weights.

Weight Lifting: Incorporating free weights or machines for exercises like deadlifts, bench presses, and leg presses helps in muscle gain. Vegan athletes can focus on high protein intake from sources like seitan, tofu, and legumes to support muscle recovery and growth.

Circuit Training: Combine short bursts of resistance exercises with minimal rest in between. For example, a circuit could include leg presses, chest presses, rows, and deadlifts, using either bodyweight or equipment like dumbbells or resistance bands. This approach helps in building muscle while also keeping the heart rate up.

.

Cardiovascular Exercises

Cardiovascular exercises are essential for heart health and endurance include:

Running or Jogging: These are excellent for cardiovascular health and can be easily incorporated into a vegan fitness plan.

Cycling: Offers a low-impact option for improving cardiovascular endurance.

Zumba or Dance Classes: Provide a fun and engaging way to incorporate cardio into your routine, boosting mood and energy levels.

Recovery and Energy Management

Post-workout nutrition is key for recovery on a vegan diet and here's why:

Protein-rich Snacks: Vegan protein bars or shakes with pea, rice, or soy protein can help in muscle repair and recovery post-workout.

Balanced Meals: Incorporating a variety of plant-based protein sources, whole grains, and healthy fats in meals throughout the day supports sustained energy levels and recovery.

These workout routines, when combined with a nutritionally rich vegan diet, ensure that individuals not only meet their fitness goals but also support their overall health and well-being.

Adapting these workout routines to fit individual fitness levels and goals, while ensuring a well-balanced vegan diet, can lead to optimal health benefits, muscle gain, and endurance improvement. It's about finding the right balance that suits your body's needs and aligns with your ethical and dietary choices.

Nutritional Strategies for Enhanced Recovery

In the realm of vegan fitness, nutritional strategies play a pivotal role in enhancing recovery post-workout. Focusing on plant-based foods and supplements can significantly reduce inflammation, speed up muscle repair, and improve overall recovery time. Here's how:

Anti-inflammatory Foods

Plant-based diets are rich in anti-inflammatory foods, which are essential for reducing inflammation caused by intense workouts. Foods such as berries, leafy greens, nuts, seeds, and whole grains are packed with antioxidants and polyphenols that help mitigate inflammation and facilitate recovery.

Protein for Muscle Repair

Protein is crucial for muscle repair and growth. Plant-based sources like tofu, tempeh, legumes, and quinoa provide the necessary amino acids for muscle synthesis. Incorporating a variety of these protein sources ensures a comprehensive amino acid profile for optimal muscle recovery.

Supplements for Enhanced Recovery

Certain supplements can complement a plant-based diet to support recovery. Omega-3 fatty acids, found in algae supplements, reduce inflammation and soreness. Vitamin B12, often supplemented in vegan diets, is vital for energy production and muscle repair. Additionally, antioxidants such as vitamins C and E, found in fruits and vegetables, further support recovery by neutralizing free radicals produced during exercise.

Hydration and Electrolytes

Staying hydrated and maintaining electrolyte balance is essential for recovery. Coconut water, rich in potassium and magnesium, and bananas, known for their high potassium content, can help replenish electrolytes lost during exercise, promoting quicker recovery and preventing muscle cramps.

By incorporating these nutritional strategies, people who are following a vegan diet can enhance their recovery process, ensuring they're ready for their next workout session with reduced downtime. This comprehensive approach not only supports physical recovery but also contributes to long-term health and wellness.

Chapter 7: Transitioning to Veganism

Transitioning to a vegan lifestyle represents a profound change in dietary practices and ethical beliefs, underscoring a dedication to the well-being of animals, the preservation of the environment, and the enhancement of personal health. This pivotal shift involves more than just modifying what one eats; it's about aligning daily choices with a broader vision of compassion and sustainability.

Recognizing the challenges this transition may present, this chapter is meticulously designed to offer a thorough roadmap for individuals embarking on this journey. Through practical advice, personal insights, and evidence-based strategies, it aims to equip readers with the tools and knowledge needed to successfully adopt and sustain a vegan lifestyle.

Addressing common hurdles such as dietary adjustments, social dynamics, and nutritional considerations, the guide emphasizes the importance of gradual change, informed choices, and self-compassion. It also shines a light on the rewards of veganism, from health benefits to a sense of global responsibility, encouraging a deep and lasting commitment to this life-affirming choice.

A Step-by-Step Guide to Adopting a Vegan Lifestyle

Initiating the vegan journey involves gradual changes rather than an overnight overhaul. Begin by eliminating one animal product at a time and gradually replacing them with plant-based alternatives. Educating oneself about vegan nutrition ensures a balanced diet while exploring diverse vegan recipes keeps meals interesting. Additionally, connecting with the vegan community online or locally can offer support and inspiration.

The journey to veganism should start with small, manageable steps to ensure a sustainable transition. Here's a structured approach to adopting a vegan lifestyle:

Eliminate Animal Products Gradually: Instead of going vegan overnight, start by cutting out one animal product at a time. This could be beginning with the easiest for you to give up and gradually moving to more challenging items. This method helps in adjusting both your palate and your cooking habits to a plant-based regime without feeling overwhelmed.

Educate Yourself: Knowledge is power, especially when transitioning to a lifestyle that is quite different from what you might be used to. Spend time learning about vegan nutrition to ensure you are getting a balanced diet. Understanding the nutritional content of plant-based foods and how to get essential nutrients like protein, iron, calcium, and vitamins will help you maintain good health throughout your transition.

Explore Vegan Recipes: One of the joys of veganism is discovering a wide array of dishes that are both nutritious and flavorful. Dive into vegan recipes and cooking techniques to keep your meals interesting and varied. This exploration not only makes your diet enjoyable but also expands your culinary skills.

Connect with the Vegan Community: Whether online or in your local area, connecting with fellow vegans can greatly enhance your transition experience. The vegan community can offer support, inspiration, and practical advice. Sharing experiences and challenges with others who have gone through or are going through a similar transition can be incredibly motivating.

By following these steps, transitioning to a vegan lifestyle can be a fulfilling and enriching journey. Remember, the shift to veganism is not just about what you're giving up but also about the new foods, flavors, and communities you're embracing.

Overcoming Challenges and Staying Committed

To overcome challenges and stay committed to a vegan lifestyle, it's crucial to have a clear understanding of your motivations, whether they are related to health, ethics, or environmental sustainability. Here's how to navigate these challenges effectively:

Identify Your Motivation: Reflect on why you chose to pursue a vegan lifestyle. Is it to improve your health, for ethical reasons concerning animal welfare, or to reduce environmental impact? Keeping these reasons in mind can help you stay focused and committed even when faced with challenges.

Stay up to date: Dive deep into vegan nutrition to make sure you're hitting all your dietary marks. This deep dive will arm you with the info you need to confidently tackle any questions or concerns others might have about your eating habits.

Build a Support System: Connect with the vegan community, either online or locally. Sharing experiences, challenges, and successes with like-minded individuals can provide encouragement and motivation.

Develop Coping Strategies: Anticipate potential social situations or dietary challenges and prepare strategies to address them. This could include bringing your own food to social events or having a list of vegan-friendly restaurants.

Celebrate Your Choices: Remember that each meal is an opportunity to reaffirm your commitment to your values. Celebrate the positive impact your choices have on your health, animals, and the planet.

By understanding your motivations, educating yourself on vegan nutrition, building a supportive community, preparing for challenges, and celebrating your choices, you can effectively overcome obstacles and maintain a long-term commitment to veganism.

Finding Vegan Alternatives and Eating Out

Adopting a vegan lifestyle opens up a world of culinary exploration, enabling you to enjoy your favorite foods with plant-based alternatives. The key to successfully dining out as a vegan and finding satisfying alternatives lies in preparation and flexibility.

Research Restaurants: Before dining out, research restaurants to find those offering vegan options or are willing to accommodate vegan diets. Websites and apps like HappyCow provide a comprehensive list of vegan and vegan-friendly restaurants globally.

CHAPTER 7: TRANSITIONING TO VEGANISM

Understanding Menu Items: Learn to identify non-vegan ingredients hidden in dishes. Ask questions about the ingredients and preparation methods to ensure your meals are vegan.

Choosing the Right Places: Ethnic restaurants such as Indian, Middle Eastern, Thai, and Ethiopian often have naturally vegan dishes due to the cultural reliance on plant-based ingredients.

Exploring Vegan Alternatives: Many traditional dishes have delicious vegan versions. Explore grocery stores, health food stores, and online resources for vegan alternatives to your favorite foods. Experiment with plant-based ingredients to recreate beloved dishes at home.

Adapting to a vegan lifestyle does not mean sacrificing the joy of eating out or enjoying your favorite meals. With a bit of planning and creativity, you can navigate any dining situation while staying true to your vegan principles.

Chapter 8: Meal Planning and Prep

Alright, let's dive into Chapter 8, where we're all about getting you set up for success in the vegan kitchen. Think of this chapter as your go-to guide for making meal planning and prep not just doable, but totally enjoyable. We're here to arm you with all the know-how you need to keep your diet full of variety, nutrition, and, of course, deliciousness, no matter how packed your schedule is.

We get it, life's busy and sometimes, figuring out what to eat can feel like just another task on an endless to-do list. But, we're flipping the script! This chapter is packed with practical tips and tricks to help you manage your kitchen like a pro, ensuring you've always got something tasty and nourishing to eat. From stocking up on essential pantry staples to whipping up meals that'll make your taste buds dance, we've got you covered.

So, if you're ready to make your vegan meal planning and prep a breeze while keeping everything nutritious and balanced, you're in the right place. Let's make your kitchen adventures as smooth and stress-free as possible, shall we?

CHAPTER 8: MEAL PLANNING AND PREP

Essential Pantry Items and How to Stock a Vegan Kitchen

To kick off your vegan kitchen adventure, let's zero in on the must-haves that'll be the backbone of your cooking.Creating a well-stocked vegan pantry is your first step towards a seamless and enjoyable cooking experience. Let's break down the must-haves:

Legumes: Beans, lentils, chickpeas, and peas are not only protein-packed but also versatile. They're great in everything from salads to soups.

Grains: Quinoa, rice, barley, and oats offer essential carbs and fiber. They're perfect as meal bases or sides.

Nuts and Seeds: Almonds, cashews, flaxseeds, and chia seeds bring in healthy fats, protein, and a crunch to meals or snacks.

Plant-Based Milks: Almond, soy, oat, and coconut milk are great for cereals, baking, or just to enjoy as a drink.

Spices and Condiments: Stock up on your favorites to add flavor to any dish. Don't forget nutritional yeast for that cheesy flavor!

Essential Oils and Vinegars: Olive oil, coconut oil, balsamic, and apple cider vinegar are great for cooking and dressings.

With these staples, you're well on your way to creating delicious, nutritious vegan meals at a moment's notice. Remember, variety is key to a balanced diet, so explore and experiment with different items to keep your meals interesting and wholesome.

Sample Meal Plans and Prep Tips for Busy Individuals

For those with a packed schedule, diving into a vegan lifestyle doesn't have to mean hours spent in the kitchen. This part of the chapter is all about making your life easier with sample meal plans designed for various needs and practical prep tips for the busy bee.

Sample Meal Plans

Quick Weekday Dinners: These plans are perfect when you've got minimal time but crave something hearty. Think 15-minute pasta dishes, stir-fries, and one-pan wonders that are as satisfying as they are quick to whip up.

Meal Prep for the Workweek: Here, we lay out how to spend a couple of hours over the weekend preparing meals that'll last you through the workweek. From bulk-cooking grains and legumes to prepping veggies, we've got you covered.

Nutritious Meals on a Budget: Eating vegan doesn't have to break the bank. These meal plans focus on affordable ingredients like beans, lentils, rice, and seasonal produce to create delicious, nutrient-packed meals.

Prep Tips for Efficiency

Batch Cooking: Cooking in large quantities can save you tons of time. Think big pots of soups, stews, or chili that can be enjoyed throughout the week or frozen for later.

Creative Leftovers: We'll show you how to transform last night's dinner into today's lunch with a twist. Leftover veggies can become a vibrant stir-fry and that batch of beans? Perfect for taco fillings or hearty salads.

Planning Ahead: A little planning goes a long way. We offer strategies for mapping out your meals for the week, making grocery shopping more straightforward, and ensuring you always have something ready to go when hunger strikes.

Armed with these plans and tips, you're all set to tackle your busy week while enjoying a variety of vegan meals that are not just convenient but also packed with flavor and nutrients.

Navigating Nutritional Balance and Variety

In the realm of vegan meal planning and prep, ensuring your diet is nutritionally comprehensive is key. This part zeroes in on the strategies to weave a rich tapestry of nutrients through your meals, ensuring you hit all the right notes with macronutrients (proteins, carbs, and fats) and crucial micronutrients (like vitamins B12 and D, iron, and calcium) that sometimes get missed in vegan diets.

Diversity is your best friend here. By including a variety of fruits, vegetables, whole grains, nuts, seeds, and legumes in your meals, you're not just adding colors to your plate but ensuring that you're covering the full spectrum of necessary nutrients. This variety is crucial for bolstering overall health and averting the common nutritional pitfalls of a vegan diet. Here's how to keep your meals diverse and nutritious:

Diversify Your Plate: Aim to include a colorful array of vegetables, fruits, grains, and protein sources in every meal. This not only makes your plate more appealing but also ensures you're getting a wide range of nutrients. Think rainbow when you shop and prep!

Know Your Nutrient Sources: Familiarize yourself with plant-based sources of essential nutrients. Legumes, nuts, and seeds are fantastic for protein; leafy greens and almonds are great for calcium; lentils and tofu can boost your iron intake; and fortified foods along with supplements can help with your B12 and vitamin D levels.

Plan with Precision: Use meal plans as a tool to ensure you're covering all nutritional bases over the course of a week. Incorporating a variety of whole foods can prevent any dietary gaps.

Embrace Supplementation Wisely: While a well-planned vegan diet can meet most nutritional needs, supplements such as B12, vitamin D, and sometimes omega-3s from algae oil can provide an essential safety net.

Seek Inspiration: Keep your meal rotation exciting by exploring new recipes and cuisines. International dishes often incorporate a broad spectrum of ingredients that can enrich your diet with flavors and nutrients.

Understanding and applying these strategies can make all the difference in thriving on a vegan diet. By prioritizing nutritional balance and variety, you ensure your body receives the full spectrum of nutrients needed to support vibrant health, all while enjoying the culinary diversity that veganism has to offer.

Chapter 9: Recipes for Revival

Welcome to the chapter, where the magic of vegan cooking unfolds across every page! This chapter is your culinary companion, showcasing a plethora of nutritious vegan recipes that cater to every meal of the day. We're diving deep into the vibrant world of vegan cuisine, with a keen eye on raw and high-protein dishes that promise to bolster your health and wellness journey.

From the break of dawn with energizing breakfasts to the tranquil end of the day with satisfying dinners, we've got you covered. And let's not forget about those essential in-between moments – our lunches and snacks ensure you're fueled and ready to tackle anything that comes your way.

Breakfasts, Lunches, Dinners, and Snacks for Optimal Health

This section is all about fueling your body with the best of vegan goodness. Whether you're kick-starting your day, searching for that perfect lunch, sitting down to a comforting dinner, or just in need of a snack, we've got you covered with recipes that are not only delicious but also packed with nutritional value. Here's what we've lined up for you:

Breakfasts

Begin your day on a high note with energy-boosting meals. Think smoothie bowls bursting with fruits, nuts, and seeds, or savory options like tofu scramble wraps loaded with veggies. These recipes are designed to provide sustained energy throughout the morning.

- **maple syrup for sweetness**. Cook on a non-stick pan until golden brown. Serve with fresh berries and a drizzle of maple syrup.
- **Tofu Scramble:** Sauté crumbled tofu with turmeric for color, nutritional yeast for a cheesy flavor, and your favorite veggies like spinach, mushrooms, and tomatoes. Season with salt and pepper.
- **Smoothie Bowls**: Blend bananas, mixed berries, and plant-based milk or yogurt until smooth. Pour into a bowl and top with sliced fruits, nuts, seeds, and a handful of granola for crunch.

Lunches: For lunch, we're keeping things vibrant and nutritious. Salads that go beyond the basics, incorporating grains like quinoa for that extra protein punch, Suchi and wraps filled with an array of colorful veggies and rich, creamy dressings.

- **Chickpea Salad Sandwich**: Mash chickpeas and mix with vegan

CHAPTER 9: RECIPES FOR REVIVAL

mayo, diced celery, red onion, and a squeeze of lemon juice. Season with salt and pepper, then serve on toasted whole-grain bread with lettuce.

- **Vegan Sushi Rolls**: Prepare sushi rice according to package instructions. On a nori sheet, layer rice, thin slices of cucumber, carrot, bell pepper, and avocado. Roll tightly and slice into sushi pieces.
- **Quinoa Salad**: Combine cooked quinoa with black beans, corn, diced tomatoes, avocado, and cilantro. Dress with lime juice, olive oil, salt, and pepper for a refreshing and filling salad.

Dinners

Evening meals are all about comfort without compromise. Dive into hearty stews, innovative plant-based takes on classic dishes, and pasta loaded with seasonal vegetables. These dinners are not just satisfying; they're also wholesome.

- **Vegan Chili:** Cook onions, garlic, and bell peppers until soft. Add canned tomatoes, kidney beans, black beans, corn, and chilli powder. Simmer until flavorful. Serve with avocado and fresh cilantro.
- **Lentil Bolognese:** Sauté onions, carrots, and celery. Add lentils, canned tomatoes, and Italian herbs. Simmer until the lentils are tender. Serve over your favorite pasta or zucchini noodles.
- **Stuffed Bell Peppers**: Mix cooked rice, black beans, corn, salsa, and vegan cheese. Stuff into halved bell peppers and bake until the peppers are tender. Top with avocado slices and fresh cilantro.

Snacks

Snack time doesn't have to be a nutritional afterthought. Enjoy snacks that keep you going without weighing you down, from homemade energy bars and fruit leathers to crispy kale chips and nutty trail mixes.

- **Energy Balls**: Combine oats, flaxseed, peanut butter, maple syrup, and vegan chocolate chips in a bowl. Roll into balls and refrigerate until firm.
- **Kale Chips:** Toss kale leaves in a bit of olive oil and your choice of seasoning. Bake in a preheated oven until crispy.
- **Hummus and Veggie Sticks:** Blend chickpeas, tahini, lemon juice, and garlic until smooth. Serve with carrot sticks, cucumber, and bell pepper slices

Each recipe within this section is carefully curated to ensure you're getting a wide range of nutrients while enjoying the flavors you love. Embrace the diversity of vegan cuisine and discover how every meal can contribute to your health and well-being.

Special Focus on Raw and High Protein Vegan Meals

A raw vegan diet is not only about eliminating animal products from your diet but also about emphasizing the consumption of uncooked and unprocessed plant-based foods. Here are some of the health benefits associated with following a raw vegan diet:

Improved heart health: Consuming raw fruits, vegetables, nuts, and seeds can lead to lower levels of cholesterol and triglycerides, reducing the risk of heart disease.

Weight loss and management: A raw vegan diet is typically low in calories and high in fiber, which can help in losing weight and maintaining a healthy weight. The high fiber content also promotes satiety, reducing overall calorie intake.

Enhanced digestive health: The high intake of dietary fiber from fruits and vegetables can improve digestion and prevent issues such as constipation. Raw foods also contain enzymes that aid in the digestion process.

Improved skin health: Many people on a raw vegan diet report clearer, more radiant skin. This could be due to the high intake of vitamins, minerals, and antioxidants that combat inflammation and oxidative stress, leading to healthier skin.

Increased energy levels: Those following a raw vegan diet often report higher energy levels, which could be attributed to the consumption of nutrient-dense, natural foods that are easily metabolized by the body.

Lower risk of chronic diseases: A raw vegan diet can lower the risk of developing chronic conditions such as type 2 diabetes, certain cancers, and other inflammatory diseases due to its high content of antioxidants and anti-inflammatory foods.

While a raw vegan diet offers numerous health benefits, it's important to ensure it is well-planned to meet all nutritional needs, particularly in terms of protein, vitamins B12 and D, iron, and calcium. Consulting with a healthcare professional or a dietitian can help ensure that you're receiving a balanced intake of all essential nutrients.

Raw Vegan Recipes

Zucchini Noodles with Avocado Pesto: Spiralized zucchini noodles tossed in a creamy avocado pesto sauce, offering a raw meal that's both nutritious and satisfying.

Ingredients:

- 2 large zucchinis, spiralized
- 1 ripe avocado
- 1/2 cup fresh basil leaves
- 2 cloves garlic
- 2 tbsp lemon juice
- 1/4 cup pine nuts or walnuts
- Salt and pepper, to taste
- Cherry tomatoes for garnish

Instructions:

- Blend the avocado, basil, garlic, lemon juice, nuts, salt, and pepper until smooth to make the pesto.
- Toss the spiralized zucchini in the avocado pesto until well coated.
- Serve garnished with cherry tomatoes.

Raw Taco Wraps: Walnut meat, avocado, fresh salsa, and cashew sour cream wrapped in crisp lettuce leaves for a raw take on taco night.

Ingredients:

- 1 cup walnuts, soaked for 2-4 hours

- 1 tsp cumin
- 1/2 tsp garlic powder
- 1/2 tsp chili powder
- 1 ripe avocado, sliced
- 1/2 cup fresh salsa
- 1/2 cup cashews, soaked for 2-4 hours (for cashew sour cream)
- Lemon juice, water, and salt (for cashew sour cream)
- Crisp lettuce leaves

Instructions:

- Process the soaked walnuts with cumin, garlic powder, and chili powder until a "meaty" texture is achieved.
- Blend the soaked cashews with lemon juice, water, and salt to taste until smooth for the sour cream.
- Assemble the tacos using lettuce leaves as the wrap, filled with walnut meat, avocado slices, fresh salsa, and a dollop of cashew sour cream.

Raw Berry Cheesecake: A no-bake cheesecake with a nutty crust and a creamy cashew and berry filling, proving that desserts can be both raw and decadent.

Ingredients:

- For the crust: 1 cup almonds, 1 cup dates
- For the filling: 2 cups cashews (soaked for 4-6 hours), 1 cup mixed berries, 1/2 cup maple syrup, 1/4 cup coconut oil, melted
- For the topping: Fresh berries

Instructions:

- Process almonds and dates until sticky and press into the bottom of a springform pan.
- Blend the soaked cashews, berries, maple syrup, and coconut oil until smooth and creamy. Pour over the crust.
- Refrigerate for at least 4 hours or until set. Garnish with fresh berries before serving.

Protein-Packed Green Smoothie: A nourishing blend of leafy greens, protein powder, and fruit, perfect for energy and muscle recovery.

Ingredients:

- 2 cups spinach
- 1 banana
- 1/2 avocado
- 2 tbsp hemp seeds
- 1 tbsp chia seeds
- 1 cup almond milk

Instructions:

- Blend all ingredients until smooth. Enjoy immediately for a protein boost.

Almond Butter Protein Balls: a nutritious snack combining almond butter, oats, protein powder, and honey for a quick energy boost and muscle repair.

Ingredients:

- 1 cup oats

CHAPTER 9: RECIPES FOR REVIVAL

- 1/2 cup almond butter
- 1/4 cup hemp seeds
- 1/4 cup maple syrup
- 1 tsp vanilla extract

Instructions:

- Mix all ingredients in a bowl. Roll into balls and refrigerate until firm.

Spirulina Energy Balls: Power-packed snack with spirulina, nuts, and dates, offering antioxidants, protein, and a natural energy boost.

Ingredients:

- 1 cup dates, pitted
- 1/2 cup almonds
- 1/2 cup walnuts
- 2 tablespoons spirulina powder
- 1 tablespoon chia seeds
- 1 tablespoon flaxseed meal
- Desiccated coconut or cocoa powder for coating

Instructions:

- In a food processor, blend the almonds and walnuts until they reach a coarse meal consistency.
- Add the pitted dates, spirulina powder, chia seeds, and flaxseed meal to the processor. Blend until the mixture starts to stick together.
- Take small amounts of the mixture and roll into balls.
- Roll the balls in desiccated coconut or cocoa powder for an extra

layer of flavor and texture.
- Place the energy balls in the refrigerator for at least an hour to firm up before serving.

These Spirulina Energy Balls are perfect as a high-protein snack, offering a burst of energy and a wealth of nutrients. Spirulina is known for its high protein content and array of vitamins and minerals, making these balls an ideal addition to a raw vegan diet.

These examples are just the tip of the iceberg. The beauty of a vegan diet, especially when exploring raw and high-protein meals, is the incredible variety and the endless combinations you can experiment with. Whether you're whipping up a quick smoothie bowl loaded with seeds and nuts for breakfast, tossing together a bean salad for lunch, or enjoying a hearty lentil stew for dinner, the options are limitless. And the best part? You're nourishing your body with every bite while keeping things delicious. So go ahead, explore, and enjoy the journey of discovering new favorites in the vegan kitchen!

Diving into a raw vegan diet can be a game changer for your health! It's like giving your body a natural detox while still enjoying a rainbow of foods. Imagine biting into fresh, crunchy salads, sipping on vibrant green smoothies, and indulging in sweet fruit platters - all while your body says a big 'thank you' by shedding unwanted pounds, revving up your energy levels, and making your skin glow like never before. Plus, waving goodbye to processed foods means you're less likely to run into pesky health issues like high blood pressure or type 2 diabetes. It's not just about eating your veggies; it's about unlocking a more vibrant, healthier you!

These benefits, ranging from physical health improvements to mental well-being, showcase the potential positive impacts of a raw vegan diet.

Seasonal and Festive Vegan Recipes

Let's dive into the world of festive vegan cooking, where we can celebrate the seasons and special occasions with dishes that are as nourishing as they are delicious. Here are a few recipes to get the holiday spirit going, showcasing not just the versatility of vegan ingredients but also their health benefits.

Vegan Roast "Turkey"

Ingredients:

A blend of vital wheat gluten and chickpea flour for the base, seasoned with sage, rosemary, and thyme for that classic holiday flavor, and stuffed with a savory mix of sautéed mushrooms, onions, garlic, and breadcrumbs.

Health Benefits:

Chickpea flour is rich in protein and fiber, supporting muscle health and digestive wellness. Mushrooms provide a source of antioxidants and vitamins D and B.

Approach:

Mix vital wheat gluten and chickpea flour with herbs to create a dough. Sauté mushrooms, onions, and garlic for the stuffing. Wrap the stuffing with the dough, shape into a loaf, and bake until golden.

Festive Cranberry-Pear Sauce

Ingredients:

Fresh cranberries and ripe pears simmered with a touch of orange zest and a cinnamon stick.

Health Benefits:

Cranberries are packed with vitamins C and E, antioxidants, and fiber, helping to support the immune system and reduce inflammation. Pears add additional fiber for digestive health.

Approach:

Combine cranberries, diced pears, orange zest, and a cinnamon stick in a saucepan. Simmer until the cranberries burst and the sauce thickens. Cool before serving.

Winter Squash and Black Bean Enchiladas

Ingredients:

Roasted winter squash and black beans wrapped in corn tortillas, smothered in a homemade enchilada sauce and baked to perfection.

Health Benefits:

Winter squash is a great source of vitamins A and C, promoting eye health and immunity, while black beans are high in protein and iron, which are essential for energy and overall health.

CHAPTER 9: RECIPES FOR REVIVAL

Approach:

Roast cubed winter squash until tender. Mix with black beans and roll in corn tortillas. Pour homemade enchilada sauce over the top and bake until bubbly.

Creamy Vegan Eggnog

Ingredients:

A rich blend of soaked cashews, coconut milk, Medjool dates, and traditional eggnog spices such as nutmeg and cinnamon, all blended until smooth.

Health Benefits:

Cashews are a heart-healthy fat source that can help lower bad cholesterol levels. Coconut milk provides medium-chain triglycerides (MCTs), known for their energy-boosting properties.

Approach:

Blend soaked cashews, coconut milk, medjool dates, and spices until smooth. Chill and serve with a sprinkle of nutmeg on top.

Spiced Pumpkin Pie

Ingredients:

A silky pumpkin filling made with pureed pumpkin, tofu, maple syrup, and a warm spice blend, all in a crispy vegan pastry crust.

Health Benefits:

Pumpkin is a low-calorie vegetable rich in beta-carotene, which the body converts into vitamin A, crucial for healthy skin and vision. Tofu adds a punch of plant-based protein.

Approach:

Blend pumpkin puree, silken tofu, maple syrup, and spices until smooth. Pour into a vegan pastry crust and bake until set. Cool before serving.

Gingerbread Cookies

Ingredients:

A mix of whole wheat and almond flour, molasses, ginger, cinnamon, and cloves, cut into festive shapes and baked.

Health Benefits:

Almond flour offers a good source of vitamin E and magnesium, while ginger provides anti-inflammatory benefits and aids in digestion.

Approach:

Mix flour, molasses, spices, and a binding agent to form a dough. Roll out, cut into shapes, and bake until crisp.

These recipes are just a starting point to explore the richness of vegan cooking during the holidays and beyond. Each ingredient brings not only flavor but also a host of health benefits, making every meal a celebration

CHAPTER 9: RECIPES FOR REVIVAL

of well-being and joy.

Remember, vegan cooking is all about experimentation and personalization, so feel free to adjust spices and ingredients to match your taste preferences and nutritional needs!

Chapter 10: Sustaining Your Vegan Lifestyle

Welcome to a pivotal chapter in your vegan journey. Here, we explore the essence of sustaining a vegan lifestyle, not just as a diet but as a holistic approach to living. It's about harmonizing your choices with your deepest values for health, wellness, and environmental care. This chapter is your compass, guiding you through practical strategies, and providing the encouragement you need to thrive on this path.

Embracing veganism is a profound commitment to yourself, the planet, and all its inhabitants. It's a lifestyle that challenges conventional choices and invites you to live with intention and compassion. We understand that this journey comes with its unique set of challenges, from navigating social situations to finding joy in vegan cooking and eating. That's why this chapter is dedicated to equipping you with the knowledge, skills, and inspiration to sustain your vegan lifestyle over the long haul.

Remember, every meal, every decision, and every step forward on this path contributes to a healthier body, a more sustainable planet, and a kinder world. Let's embark on this journey together, with confidence and joy, knowing that the choices we make today shape a better tomorrow for all beings.

CHAPTER 10: SUSTAINING YOUR VEGAN LIFESTYLE

Navigating Social Situations and Dining Out

Heading out to eat and worried about sticking to your vegan lifestyle? Don't sweat it! Eating vegan at any restaurant is totally doable—and nope, you won't be stuck munching on just salad (unless you're into that). So, what's the game plan?

First off, let's talk about those hidden gems on the menu. Many spots might surprise you with vegan-friendly starters like crispy fried pickles, those irresistible sweet potato fries, or even a hearty vegetable chili. And BBQ veggies? Yes, please! Sometimes, you might even stumble upon some BBQ tofu.

Now, when you're planning to dine out, a little research goes a long way. Checking out the restaurant's menu online beforehand can give you a heads-up on what vegan options they have. And if the menu isn't clear, just give them a ring! Most places are more than happy to chat about their dishes and how they can accommodate your vegan needs.

Finding vegan options while dining out is becoming easier than ever! A little preparation and a conversation with the restaurant staff can effortlessly align your dining experience with your vegan lifestyle. So, go ahead and relish your meal with ease and joy!

In a nutshell,

- **Communicate Your Needs:** Don't hesitate to share your dietary preferences with hosts or restaurant staff. Most are willing to accommodate your needs.
- **Plan Ahead**: Research restaurants in advance to ensure they offer vegan options. When attending social events, consider eating

beforehand or bringing a dish to share.
- **Focus on Inclusivity**: Remember, social events are about connecting with others. Keep the focus on the company, not just the food.

Long-term Strategies for Maintaining Your Vegan Journey

Heading into the world of veganism can feel like you're navigating a maze without a map, especially when it comes to social situations. Ever been to a dinner where the only "vegan" option was a sad side salad? Or tried explaining your dietary choices without sounding like you're giving a lecture? It's all part of the adventure.

Here's the lowdown: dining out or attending family gatherings doesn't have to be a sweat-inducing ordeal. It's all about having a game plan. Before hitting the town, do a little homework to find vegan-friendly spots. Most places are more than willing to accommodate if you give them a heads-up. And when you're a guest, bringing a vegan dish to share not only guarantees you something yummy to eat but also opens up a conversation about veganism without the preachy vibe.

Remember, being vegan is about making choices that feel right to you, not about being perfect. So, if you accidentally eat something non-vegan, don't beat yourself up. It's about the journey, not the destination. And who knows? Your positive approach might just inspire someone else to give veganism a try.

CHAPTER 10: SUSTAINING YOUR VEGAN LIFESTYLE

Encouragement to Embark on the Vegan Journey for Health, Wellness, and Environmental Reasons

Diving into veganism isn't just about swapping steak for tofu; it's about embarking on a journey that's kind to your body, the planet, and all its inhabitants. Imagine lowering your risk of some hefty health concerns like heart disease, high blood pressure, diabetes, and even some cancers. That's the power of plants for you. And it's not just about what's on your plate; it's about taking a stand against the environmental impacts of traditional diets. By choosing plant-based, you're slashing your carbon footprint and giving Mother Earth a much-needed breather.

Choosing to live vegan isn't just a diet change; it's a profound decision that echoes through your health, the environment, and how you connect with the world. The ripple effects? They're huge. Imagine lowering the risk of major hitters like heart disease, hypertension, diabetes, and even some cancers. That's the power of plants at work in your body.

But it's not just about us, right? It's also about taking a stand for our planet. Veganism slashes your carbon footprint, making a direct impact on reducing climate change. It's about choosing kindness over convenience, compassion over indifference.

And guess what? It's absolutely doable. This isn't about perfection; it's about making choices that align more closely with your values every day. Whether you're navigating dining out, finding community support, or exploring the vast world of vegan cooking, remember: that every small choice adds up to a big difference.

So, let's dive into this journey together, equipped with the knowledge, tools, and heart to make it not just manageable but truly fulfilling. Here's to a lifestyle that celebrates health, champions the environment, and embraces compassion. Welcome to the vegan way – where every step forward is a step towards a better world for all.

Health and wellness benefits

The health benefits of adopting a vegan diet are significant and supported by scientific research. Here's a specific breakdown:

Weight Loss: Many people experience a reduction in body weight when switching to a vegan diet, attributed to lower calorie intake from plant-based foods.

Heart Health: A vegan diet can help improve heart health by lowering cholesterol levels, reducing blood pressure, and decreasing the risk of heart disease.

Diabetes Management: Vegan diets can help lower blood sugar levels and improve kidney function, which can be beneficial for managing diabetes.

Cancer Risk: Certain types of cancer, such as colon cancer, may be less likely in individuals following a vegan diet due to a higher intake of fruits, vegetables, and fiber.

Lower Blood Pressure: Plant-based diets are associated with lower blood pressure, reducing the risk of hypertension.

Improved Cholesterol Levels: Vegan diets can lead to lower levels of harmful LDL cholesterol and higher levels of beneficial HDL cholesterol.

Nutrient Intake: Despite common misconceptions, a well-planned vegan diet can provide all necessary nutrients, including fiber, vitamins, and minerals, by focusing on whole foods like fruits, vegetables, pulses, grains, nuts, and seeds.

These benefits underscore the positive impact a vegan diet can have on overall health and well-being.

Environmental Impact

Diving into veganism? That's not just good news for your health but a big win for our planet too! You see, by choosing plant-based grub over meat and dairy, you're basically giving Mother Earth a high five. Here's the lowdown: munching on veggies, grains, and all that good plant stuff significantly slashes the greenhouse gases that livestock farming belches out. We're talking about a massive reduction in your carbon footprint—up to 73% less, believe it or not!

But wait, there's more. Veganism is like hitting the eco-friendly jackpot. It drastically cuts down on the water and land needed for farming animals. Imagine, a global shift to vegan eating could shrink the land we use for agriculture by a whopping 75%. That's a lot of space for nature to do its thing, grow forests, and support biodiversity. Plus, it eases the pressure on our precious water resources.

So, in a nutshell, opting for a vegan diet is like choosing to walk lightly on the earth. It's about eating in a way that supports our health and lets the planet breathe easier. And hey, who wouldn't want to be part of that positive change? Let's keep the conversation going and spread the word about the green power of veganism!

Ethical Considerations

Jumping into veganism isn't just about munching on veggies or dodging dairy and meat; it's a big-hearted move towards living more ethically. Imagine making choices every day that help reduce animal suffering and exploitation. That's veganism in a nutshell! It's about saying "no thanks" to practices that harm animals and choosing a path of compassion instead.

By picking plant-based foods, you're taking a stand against the industrial-scale use of animals for food. It's a way of voting with your fork for a kinder world. Whether it's skipping that cheeseburger for a veggie burger or opting for almond milk over cow's milk, every choice adds up to a big statement: animals are not ours to use and abuse.

So, when you're whipping up your next meal or grocery shopping, remember you're part of a growing movement that values ethical living. It's about making choices that feel right in your heart, supporting a future where we treat all beings with respect and kindness. Let's keep the conversation going and spread the word about the compassionate, ethical side of veganism. It's not just good for the animals and our conscience; it's a step towards a more just and ethical world.

Conclusion: Your Vegan Body Revival

And there we have it! The grand finale of our plant-based adventure. From the whys to the hows, we've dived deep into what it means to embrace a vegan lifestyle—not just as a diet, but as a compassionate way of living that reverberates through every choice we make.

We've explored the myriad benefits, from the undeniable health perks to the profound environmental impact and the ethical stand against animal exploitation. It's clear that veganism is more than just a trend; it's a sustainable lifestyle that's gaining momentum across the globe. And you, my friend, are now equipped with all the tools, knowledge, and inspiration to make this lifestyle your own.

But don't let the journey end here. As you continue to explore the vast and vibrant world of veganism, remember that every meal, every purchase, and every conversation is an opportunity to advocate for a kinder, greener, and healthier planet. Your choices have power, and your voice can inspire change.

In closing, remember that veganism isn't about perfection; it's about making conscious choices that align with your values. There will be challenges and learning curves, but also joy, discovery, and a sense of fulfilment like no other. Here's to your vegan body revival and to being part of a movement that's reshaping the world, one plant-based choice at a time. Cheers to a healthier you and a happier planet!

Now, I'd love to hear from you! If this book has sparked something inside you, lit the path to veganism, or even just planted a seed of curiosity, head over to Amazon and share your thoughts. Your feedback not only supports me but also guides others who might be on the fence about leaping veganism. Plus, who doesn't love a good review?

References:

OpenAI. (2023). ChatGPT: Version [GPT 4]. Retrieved from [https://chat.openai.com/]

Printed in Great Britain
by Amazon

71cd3ecc-194f-4d7c-b5a4-b7b4f1693b98R01